Massage and Mindfulness

A Comprehensive Guide to Wellness through the Body-Mind Connection and Integrating Massage and Mindfulness for Holistic Health

Elise Little

Table of Contents

Introduction:

In our fast-paced world, where stress and anxiety often feel like constant companions, finding pathways to holistic health has never been more essential. "Massage and Mindfulness: A Comprehensive Guide to Wellness through the Body-Mind Connection" invites you on a transformative journey to explore the profound intersection of massage therapy and mindfulness practices, revealing how they can work together to nurture both body and mind.

This book is more than a guide; it is a roadmap to a richer, more balanced life. Through the lens of the body-mind connection, we will delve into the science and art of massage therapy and mindfulness, uncovering how these practices can harmonize to promote overall wellness. By integrating these two powerful tools, we can unlock new dimensions of healing and self-care, paving the way for a healthier, more fulfilled existence.

Massage therapy has long been celebrated for its physical benefits—from reducing muscle tension and alleviating pain to enhancing circulation and promoting relaxation. Yet, its impact extends beyond the physical realm. When combined with mindfulness—a practice of present-moment awareness and acceptance—we discover a synergistic approach that addresses the body, mind, and spirit. Mindfulness helps us cultivate a deeper understanding of our internal states, fostering emotional resilience and mental clarity.

In the following pages, we will explore the principles and techniques of massage therapy and mindfulness. You will learn about the various forms of massage, from Swedish and deep tissue to aromatherapy and shiatsu, and how each can be applied to support physical and emotional well-being. We will also delve into mindfulness practices, including meditation, breathing exercises, and mindful movement, and discover how they can enhance the effects of massage and vice versa.

This guide is designed to be both practical and accessible, offering step-by-step instructions, expert insights, and real-life applications. Whether you are new to massage and mindfulness or an experienced practitioner seeking to deepen your practice, you will find valuable tools and inspiration to enrich your journey toward holistic health.

Ultimately, "Massage and Mindfulness" aims to empower you to take charge of your well-being, fostering a harmonious balance between body and mind. By embracing the integration of these transformative practices, you will embark on a path of profound healing and personal growth, discovering a renewed sense of vitality and inner peace.

Welcome to a journey of holistic wellness—one where the art of massage and the practice of mindfulness converge to create a life of balance, harmony, and profound well-being.

Chapter 1: The Body-Mind Connection

The body-mind connection is a profound and intricate relationship that underlies our overall health and well-being. This concept reflects the understanding that our physical and mental states are deeply interwoven, influencing and affecting each other in ways that are both visible and subtle. At its core, the body-mind connection emphasizes that our physical sensations, emotions, thoughts, and behaviors are not separate entities but rather part of a cohesive, interactive system.

Historically, the mind-body link has been explored through various cultural and philosophical lenses. Ancient practices such as yoga, Tai Chi, and traditional Chinese medicine have long acknowledged the connection between physical health and mental states. In contemporary science, this connection is supported by research in fields like psychoneuroimmunology and neuroplasticity, which study how our mental and emotional experiences can impact our physical health.

Physiologically, the body-mind connection operates through multiple pathways. The central nervous system, including the brain and spinal cord, communicates with every organ and tissue through a complex network of neurons and neurotransmitters. This communication means that stress, anxiety, and other mental states can trigger physical responses in the body, such as increased heart rate, muscle tension, and changes in immune function. Conversely, physical experiences, such as pain or relaxation, can influence our emotional and mental states, demonstrating a bidirectional flow between body and mind.

One significant aspect of the body-mind connection is the role of stress. Chronic stress, for example, has been shown to have far-reaching effects on physical health, contributing to conditions such as hypertension, cardiovascular disease, and gastrointestinal issues. The stress response involves the release of stress hormones like cortisol, which can disrupt normal bodily functions when elevated for extended periods. On the other hand, practices that promote relaxation, such as mindfulness and massage, can counteract these effects by activating the parasympathetic nervous system, which helps restore balance and promote healing.

The psychological dimension of the body-mind connection is equally compelling. Emotions such as fear, joy, and sadness are not merely mental experiences but are felt physically in the body. For instance, anxiety might manifest as tightness in the chest, while happiness might bring about a sense of lightness and energy. Recognizing this interplay helps us understand that emotional well-being is crucial to physical health and that addressing one aspect can positively impact the other.

Integrating practices that honor the body-mind connection can lead to profound improvements in overall well-being. Techniques such as mindfulness meditation and therapeutic massage are effective in enhancing this connection. Mindfulness encourages a heightened awareness of the present moment, allowing individuals to observe their thoughts and physical sensations without judgment. This awareness can lead to reduced stress and better emotional regulation. Massage therapy, by alleviating physical tension and promoting relaxation, directly impacts the body-mind connection, facilitating a state of calm that benefits both physical and emotional health.

In sum, understanding and nurturing the body-mind connection is essential for achieving holistic health. By acknowledging how our mental and physical states interact, we can adopt more effective strategies for self-care and wellness. As we explore the principles and practices of massage and mindfulness in the following chapters, we will see how harnessing this connection can lead to a more balanced and harmonious life.

1.1 Understanding the Interplay between Mind and Body

The interplay between mind and body is a dynamic and intricate relationship that influences every aspect of our health and well-being. This connection is not merely theoretical but has practical implications for how we experience and manage stress, physical health, and emotional balance. At its essence, the mind-body connection underscores the principle that mental and physical states are deeply interdependent, each influencing and shaping the other.

When we consider how thoughts and emotions affect physical health, it's evident that the mind has a tangible impact on the body. For instance, chronic stress—an emotional state characterized by prolonged anxiety or pressure—can lead to a range of physical symptoms such as headaches, muscle tension, and digestive issues. This happens because the body responds to perceived threats or stressors with a physiological reaction known as the stress response, which includes the release of stress hormones like cortisol and adrenaline. These hormones prepare the body for a "fight-or-flight" response, altering various bodily functions to cope with the stressor. If stress persists, this response can become maladaptive, contributing to long-term health problems such as hypertension, heart disease, and a weakened immune system.

Conversely, physical conditions can also affect mental states. Chronic pain or illness can lead to feelings of frustration, sadness, or even depression. The experience of physical discomfort often leads to a cycle of negative thoughts and emotional distress, which can exacerbate the sensation of pain and hinder recovery. This cycle highlights the bidirectional nature of the mind-body connection—physical health impacts emotional well-being, and emotional states can influence physical health.

One of the key aspects of understanding this interplay is recognizing how mental practices can alter physiological responses. Techniques such as mindfulness meditation demonstrate this relationship effectively. Mindfulness involves paying attention to the present moment with acceptance and without judgment. Research has shown that regular mindfulness practice can reduce stress, lower blood pressure, and improve overall health by enhancing the body's ability to manage stress and regulate emotional responses. This practice helps break the cycle of stress and its physical repercussions, promoting a state of relaxation and balance.

Similarly, physical practices can also foster mental well-being. For example, massage therapy not only alleviates muscle tension and improves circulation but also stimulates the release of endorphins—chemicals in the brain that act as natural painkillers and mood enhancers. The act of receiving a massage can induce a state of relaxation, reducing stress levels and improving mood. This demonstrates how physical interventions can positively impact mental states and vice versa.

Understanding the interplay between mind and body encourages a holistic approach to health that acknowledges the importance of both mental and physical factors. It suggests that optimal well-being requires attention to both domains and that interventions targeting one aspect can lead to improvements in the other. By exploring and embracing this interconnectedness, we can develop more effective strategies for managing stress, improving health, and enhancing overall quality of life.

In summary, the interplay between mind and body is a profound aspect of human health. Recognizing and harnessing this connection allows us to adopt a more integrated approach to wellness, addressing both physical and mental dimensions to achieve a balanced and harmonious state of well-being.

1.2 The Science behind the Body-Mind Connection

The science behind the body-mind connection reveals a complex interplay of physiological, neurological, and biochemical processes that underscore how deeply intertwined our mental and physical states are. This connection is supported by a range of scientific disciplines, including psychology, neuroscience, and immunology, which collectively shed light on how mental states can influence physical health and vice versa.

Central to understanding this connection is the role of the nervous system, particularly the brain, and its interaction with the rest of the body. The brain processes thoughts, emotions, and sensory information, sending signals throughout the body via the central nervous system and the peripheral nervous system. These signals regulate various physiological responses, including heart rate, blood pressure, and hormone release. When we experience stress or anxiety, the brain activates the body's stress response system, primarily through the hypothalamic-pituitary-adrenal (HPA) axis. This system triggers the release of stress hormones such as cortisol and adrenaline, which prepare the body to deal with perceived threats. While this response can be beneficial in short bursts, chronic activation can lead to detrimental effects on health, including inflammation, immune system suppression, and cardiovascular problems.

Neuroscience has also explored the concept of neuroplasticity, which is the brain's ability to reorganize itself by forming new neural connections throughout life. Neuroplasticity underscores the idea that mental practices such as mindfulness and meditation can physically alter brain structures and functions. For example, research has shown that mindfulness meditation can increase the density of gray matter in areas of the brain associated with emotional regulation and self-awareness. This suggests that mental training can lead to lasting changes in brain function and structure, highlighting the profound impact that mental states can have on physical health.

The immune system further illustrates the connection between mind and body. Stress and negative emotions can suppress immune function, making the body more susceptible to illness. Conversely, positive emotional states and practices such as mindfulness have been associated with enhanced immune response and faster recovery from illness. Studies have shown that mindfulness can reduce markers of inflammation, which is a key factor in many chronic diseases. This interaction between the mind and the immune system demonstrates how emotional and mental states can directly impact physical health.

The field of psychoneuroimmunology (PNI) specifically examines the interactions between psychological processes, the nervous system, and the immune system. PNI research has revealed that psychological stress can influence immune system activity through the release of stress hormones and neurotransmitters. For instance, chronic stress can lead to elevated levels of pro-inflammatory cytokines, which are associated with various health conditions, including autoimmune diseases and cancer. Understanding these mechanisms highlights the importance of managing stress and maintaining mental well-being for overall health.

In addition to these physiological and neurological aspects, the body-mind connection is also reflected in behavioral and experiential domains. Practices such as yoga, Tai Chi, and biofeedback have been shown to improve both mental and physical health, further supporting the concept of an integrated approach to wellness. These practices combine physical movement with mental focus, demonstrating how engaging both body and mind can lead to enhanced overall health and well-being.

In summary, the science behind the body-mind connection reveals a sophisticated network of physiological and psychological interactions. By understanding how mental states influence physical health and how

physical interventions can impact mental well-being, we gain valuable
insights into achieving a more holistic and integrated approach to health.

1.3 How Stress Affects Your Physical and Mental Health

Stress is a ubiquitous aspect of modern life, and its effects on both
physical and mental health are profound and multifaceted. When we
encounter stress, our bodies initiate a series of physiological and
psychological responses designed to help us cope with perceived threats
or challenges. While these responses are adaptive in the short term,
chronic or excessive stress can lead to significant health problems,
illustrating the intricate relationship between stress, physical health, and
mental well-being.

The physiological stress response involves the activation of the body's
stress response systems, primarily the hypothalamic-pituitary-adrenal
(HPA) axis and the autonomic nervous system. When a stressor is
perceived, the brain signals the adrenal glands to release stress
hormones, including cortisol and adrenaline. These hormones prepare
the body for a "fight-or-flight" response by increasing heart rate,
elevating blood pressure, and redirecting blood flow to vital organs and
muscles. While these changes are beneficial in acute situations,
prolonged activation of the stress response can have detrimental effects.

Chronic stress leads to sustained high levels of cortisol, which can
disrupt various bodily functions. One major impact is on the
cardiovascular system. Persistent stress can contribute to hypertension,
increased risk of heart disease, and stroke. Elevated cortisol levels can
cause inflammation and damage to blood vessels, promoting the
development of atherosclerosis and other cardiovascular conditions.
Additionally, stress can negatively affect the immune system, making

the body more susceptible to infections and slowing down the healing process.

Stress also has significant effects on the digestive system. Stress-induced changes in hormone levels and blood flow can lead to gastrointestinal issues such as irritable bowel syndrome (IBS), acid reflux, and ulcers. The stress response can alter gut motility and increase the production of stomach acid, contributing to these problems. Furthermore, chronic stress can impact appetite, leading to overeating or loss of appetite, which in turn affects overall nutritional status and health.

On the mental health front, stress is closely linked to emotional and cognitive difficulties. Prolonged exposure to stress can lead to anxiety and depression, as the constant activation of stress pathways affects brain function and emotional regulation. High levels of cortisol can impair the hippocampus, a brain region involved in memory and learning, resulting in difficulties with concentration, memory, and decision-making. Stress also affects mood, often leading to feelings of irritability, frustration, and helplessness.

Moreover, the psychological impact of stress can create a vicious cycle, where stress contributes to mental health issues, which in turn exacerbate the stress response. For example, anxiety can lead to heightened awareness of stressors, further increasing stress levels and negatively affecting mental well-being. This cycle can be difficult to break without intervention.

To manage stress effectively and mitigate its impact on physical and mental health, it is crucial to adopt strategies that promote relaxation and resilience. Techniques such as mindfulness meditation, physical exercise, and adequate sleep are known to help regulate the stress response and improve overall health. By addressing both the physiological and psychological aspects of stress, individuals can enhance their ability to cope with challenges and maintain a balanced state of well-being.

In summary, stress has far-reaching effects on both physical and mental health. The body's adaptive stress response becomes maladaptive when experienced chronically, leading to a range of health problems. Understanding these effects emphasizes the importance of effective stress management techniques to protect and enhance overall well-being.

Chapter 2: The Fundamentals of Massage Therapy

Massage therapy, an ancient practice with roots in various cultures, has evolved into a recognized and widely practiced method for enhancing physical and mental well-being. At its core, massage therapy involves the manipulation of the body's soft tissues, including muscles, tendons, ligaments, and fascia, to promote relaxation, alleviate pain, and improve overall health. Understanding the fundamentals of massage therapy is essential for appreciating its benefits and applications in a holistic approach to wellness.

The primary technique used in massage therapy is manual manipulation. This involves applying pressure, friction, and movement to the body's soft tissues to achieve therapeutic effects. Various techniques are employed, each with specific goals and methods. For instance, Swedish massage, one of the most popular forms, uses long, flowing strokes, kneading, and circular movements to promote relaxation and improve circulation. This technique is often used to relieve stress and muscle tension, making it ideal for those seeking general relaxation and wellness.

Deep tissue massage, in contrast, targets the deeper layers of muscle and connective tissue. By using more intense pressure and focusing on specific areas of tension, deep tissue massage aims to address chronic muscle pain, stiffness, and limited range of motion. This technique is beneficial for individuals with more persistent or severe muscular issues and is often employed by athletes and those with injuries.

Another notable technique is shiatsu, a form of Japanese massage that incorporates principles of traditional Chinese medicine. Shiatsu involves applying pressure to specific points on the body to balance energy flow, known as qi. This approach not only addresses physical discomfort but also aims to harmonize the body's energy, promoting overall health and well-being.

Massage therapy operates on several physiological principles. One key mechanism is the stimulation of the parasympathetic nervous system, which counteracts the stress response by promoting relaxation and reducing the production of stress hormones. This effect helps lower heart rate and blood pressure, fostering a state of calm and reducing the physical symptoms of stress.

Massage also enhances blood circulation, which is crucial for delivering oxygen and nutrients to tissues and removing metabolic waste products. Improved circulation supports the healing process, reduces muscle soreness, and aids in the recovery of injuries. Additionally, massage helps release endorphins, the body's natural painkillers, which contribute to a sense of well-being and pain relief.

Beyond the physical benefits, massage therapy has significant mental and emotional effects. The therapeutic touch involved in massage can evoke a sense of comfort and connection, which is beneficial for emotional health. The relaxation achieved through massage can reduce anxiety, promote better sleep, and enhance overall mood. This interplay between physical relaxation and emotional balance underscores the holistic nature of massage therapy.

The practice of massage therapy is governed by various professional standards and ethics. Practitioners are trained to assess individual needs, tailor treatments accordingly, and ensure a safe and respectful environment for clients. Certification and licensing requirements vary by region, but they generally involve comprehensive education and adherence to ethical practices.

In summary, massage therapy is a versatile and effective tool for enhancing physical and mental health. By understanding its fundamental techniques and mechanisms, we can appreciate its role in promoting relaxation, improving circulation, and supporting emotional well-being. As we continue to explore massage therapy's benefits and applications, it becomes clear that it offers a valuable component of a holistic approach to health and wellness.

2.1 History and Evolution of Massage Techniques

The history and evolution of massage techniques reflect a rich tapestry of cultural practices and scientific advancements. This therapeutic approach, involving the manipulation of soft tissues, has been utilized across diverse civilizations for thousands of years, each contributing to the development of various techniques and methodologies that we recognize today.

The origins of massage can be traced back to ancient civilizations, where it was used for both therapeutic and ritualistic purposes. In ancient China, which is often cited as one of the earliest cultures to formally document massage practices, texts such as the "Yellow Emperor's Classic of Internal Medicine," dating back to around 2700 BCE, describe various forms of body manipulation for health and healing. Traditional Chinese Medicine (TCM) incorporates massage techniques, such as tui na, which focuses on stimulating acupressure points and manipulating the body's energy (qi) to balance the flow and improve health.

In ancient India, the practice of massage is deeply intertwined with Ayurvedic medicine, a holistic system that has been practiced for over 5,000 years. Ayurvedic texts like the "Sushruta Samhita" discuss massage techniques as part of a broader therapeutic approach aimed at balancing the body's doshas (vital energies). Traditional Indian massage often involves the use of herbal oils and specific techniques designed to cleanse, invigorate, and restore balance.

Similarly, ancient Egypt also has a rich history of massage. Archaeological findings, including tomb paintings and artifacts, suggest that massage was used as a therapeutic practice and a form of relaxation. The Egyptians employed various techniques, including kneading and stroking, often integrated into rituals and daily life. The practice was valued not only for its physical benefits but also for its spiritual and ceremonial significance.

The Greeks and Romans further advanced the practice of massage. The Greek physician Hippocrates, often referred to as the "Father of Medicine," wrote about the use of massage for therapeutic purposes, advocating its benefits for muscle and joint health. In ancient Rome, massage was a popular form of treatment and relaxation, practiced by both physicians and individuals. Roman baths, or thermae, were equipped with massage rooms where techniques such as rubbing, kneading, and stretching were performed.

The Middle Ages saw a decline in the practice of massage in Europe, partly due to the rise of Christian doctrines that viewed physical indulgence with suspicion. However, the therapeutic use of massage continued in other parts of the world, including the Middle East, where scholars and practitioners preserved and expanded upon earlier knowledge.

The Renaissance period marked a resurgence of interest in the sciences and a renewed exploration of ancient texts. During this time, the practice of massage was revived in Europe, with a growing emphasis on empirical observation and anatomical understanding. Notable figures such as Per Henrik Ling, a Swedish physical therapist in the early 19th century, contributed significantly to the modern development of massage techniques. Ling's system, known as Swedish massage, became widely recognized and remains one of the most popular forms of massage practiced today.

In the 20th and 21st centuries, massage therapy has continued to evolve with the integration of new scientific knowledge and therapeutic approaches. The development of evidence-based practices has led to a better understanding of the physiological and psychological effects of massage. Contemporary massage techniques have diversified, incorporating elements from various traditions and modern innovations to address a wide range of health concerns and enhance overall well-being.

In summary, the history and evolution of massage techniques reflect a journey through ancient wisdom and scientific progress. From its origins in early civilizations to its current status as a widely practiced and scientifically validated therapy, massage has adapted and expanded, offering diverse techniques and benefits for modern health and wellness.

2.2 Types of Massage and Their Benefits

Massage therapy encompasses a variety of techniques, each designed to address different needs and promote specific aspects of physical and mental well-being. Understanding the types of massage and their benefits can help individuals select the most appropriate therapy based on their personal health goals and preferences.

Swedish massage is one of the most commonly practiced forms of massage and is known for its gentle, relaxing approach. This technique involves long, flowing strokes, kneading, circular movements, and tapping. Swedish massage aims to enhance overall relaxation, improve circulation, and ease muscle tension. It is particularly beneficial for those seeking relief from everyday stress and muscle soreness, making it a popular choice for general wellness and relaxation.

Deep tissue massage focuses on the deeper layers of muscle and connective tissue. It employs slow, deliberate strokes and deep pressure to target chronic muscle tension and adhesions. This type of massage is effective for addressing persistent pain, stiffness, and restricted movement. By working through deeper muscle layers, deep tissue massage can alleviate discomfort from injuries, improve range of motion, and promote healing. It is often sought by individuals with chronic pain conditions or those recovering from physical strain.

Another technique is shiatsu, which originates from Japan and is rooted in traditional Chinese medicine principles. Shiatsu involves applying pressure to specific points along the body's meridians or energy pathways. The goal is to balance the body's energy flow (qi) and promote overall health. Shiatsu can be beneficial for reducing stress, improving energy levels, and addressing both physical and emotional imbalances. The practice is also known for enhancing relaxation and improving the body's natural healing processes.

Thai massage is a traditional practice that combines elements of acupressure, stretching, and yoga. Performed on a mat on the floor, Thai massage involves a series of assisted stretches and rhythmic compressions. This technique aims to improve flexibility, release muscle tension, and enhance overall energy flow. Thai massage is beneficial for those seeking to increase their range of motion, alleviate muscular tightness, and experience a sense of rejuvenation and balance.

Sports massage is tailored to the needs of athletes and active individuals. It incorporates techniques from various massage styles, including Swedish and deep tissue, to address the specific demands of athletic performance. Sports massage focuses on enhancing performance, preventing injuries, and aiding in recovery. It can help reduce muscle soreness, improve flexibility, and address common issues such as muscle strain and joint discomfort.

Another popular form is aromatherapy massage, which combines the benefits of massage with essential oils. During an aromatherapy massage, essential oils are selected based on their therapeutic properties and blended with carrier oils. The scents and properties of the essential oils, such as lavender for relaxation or eucalyptus for respiratory support, enhance the massage experience and provide additional health benefits. Aromatherapy massage is known for its ability to improve mood, reduce stress, and promote emotional balance.

Hot stone massage involves the use of smooth, heated stones placed on specific areas of the body. The heat from the stones helps to relax muscles, improve circulation, and provide a deep sense of relaxation. This technique is particularly useful for relieving muscle tension, promoting overall relaxation, and soothing chronic pain.

In summary, the various types of massage offer a range of benefits tailored to different needs and preferences. Whether seeking relaxation, pain relief, improved flexibility, or enhanced overall well-being, individuals can choose from techniques such as Swedish, deep tissue, shiatsu, Thai, sports, aromatherapy, and hot stone massage. Each type provides unique therapeutic effects, contributing to a comprehensive approach to health and wellness.

2.3 How Massage Therapy Influences the Body-Mind Connection

Massage therapy plays a significant role in enhancing the body-mind connection by bridging the gap between physical sensations and mental states. This therapeutic practice involves the manipulation of soft tissues to address physical discomfort, promote relaxation, and support overall well-being. The effects of massage extend beyond the physical realm, influencing emotional and psychological health in profound ways.

One of the primary ways massage therapy impacts the body-mind connection is through its ability to activate the parasympathetic nervous system. This system is responsible for the body's "rest-and-digest" response, which counteracts the stress-induced "fight-or-flight" reaction. During a massage, the stimulation of the parasympathetic nervous system leads to a decrease in heart rate, lower blood pressure, and reduced levels of stress hormones such as cortisol. This shift towards relaxation fosters a sense of calm and helps to mitigate the physical and emotional effects of stress. As a result, individuals often experience improved mood and a greater sense of emotional balance following a massage session.

Massage therapy also promotes the release of endorphins, the body's natural painkillers. These biochemical substances interact with the brain's pain receptors to diminish the sensation of pain and induce feelings of euphoria. The release of endorphins contributes to a more positive emotional state, enhancing the overall sense of well-being and reinforcing the mind-body connection. By alleviating physical discomfort and stimulating the production of endorphins, massage therapy can effectively improve mood and mental clarity.

The therapeutic touch involved in massage therapy is another crucial aspect of its influence on the body-mind connection. Physical touch has been shown to have significant emotional and psychological effects. The act of receiving a massage can evoke feelings of safety, comfort, and connection, which are essential for emotional healing and stress reduction. For many individuals, the tactile experience of massage provides a unique form of emotional support and fosters a sense of trust and relaxation.

Additionally, massage therapy can enhance body awareness and mindfulness. During a massage, individuals are encouraged to focus on their physical sensations and become more attuned to their bodies. This heightened awareness can lead to greater mindfulness, as individuals become more conscious of their physical and emotional states. Increased body awareness can help individuals identify areas of tension, discomfort, or emotional stress that may not have been previously recognized. By addressing these areas through massage, individuals can develop a deeper understanding of their body-mind connection and take proactive steps toward achieving balance and wellness.

Massage therapy also supports emotional processing and mental health. For individuals experiencing stress, anxiety, or depression, the relaxation induced by massage can provide a respite from persistent negative thought patterns. The soothing effects of massage can help individuals shift their focus away from stressors and promote a more positive outlook. This mental break allows for emotional processing and can contribute to improved mental health and emotional resilience.

In summary, massage therapy profoundly influences the body-mind connection by promoting relaxation, enhancing mood, and fostering body awareness. Through its effects on the nervous system, biochemical responses, and emotional well-being, massage therapy helps to bridge the gap between physical sensations and mental states. By addressing both physical and psychological aspects of health, massage therapy supports a holistic approach to wellness and contributes to a balanced and harmonious state of being.

Chapter 3: The Basics of Mindfulness

Mindfulness is a practice that involves paying focused, non-judgmental attention to the present moment. Originating from ancient contemplative traditions, particularly in Buddhism, mindfulness has gained widespread recognition in contemporary psychology and wellness practices due to its profound impact on mental and physical health. Understanding the basics of mindfulness can provide valuable insights into how this practice contributes to overall well-being.

At its core, mindfulness is about cultivating an awareness of the present moment, including our thoughts, emotions, and physical sensations, without being overwhelmed or influenced by them. It involves observing these experiences with a sense of openness and acceptance, rather than reacting or getting caught up in them. This practice encourages individuals to engage with their current experiences fully and intentionally, without judgment or distraction.

One of the foundational aspects of mindfulness is the practice of focused attention. This often begins with focusing on a single point of reference, such as the breath. By directing attention to the breath, individuals can anchor themselves in the present moment, which helps to counteract the tendency to ruminate about the past or worry about the future. Focusing on the breath creates a stable and calming anchor that brings awareness back to the present whenever the mind begins to wander.

Another key component of mindfulness is non-judgmental observation. This means acknowledging and accepting thoughts and feelings as they arise, without labeling them as good or bad. Mindfulness encourages individuals to observe their inner experiences with curiosity rather than criticism. For example, if a person feels anxious, mindfulness practice involves recognizing the anxiety without reacting to it or trying to suppress it. This approach fosters a more balanced and accepting relationship with one's internal experiences.

Mindfulness practice often involves techniques such as mindful breathing, body scans, and mindful movement. Mindful breathing involves paying close attention to the sensation of the breath entering and leaving the body. Body scans involve systematically directing attention to different parts of the body to increase awareness of physical sensations and promote relaxation. Mindful movement, which can be seen in practices like yoga or Tai Chi, integrates mindful awareness with physical movement, enhancing both physical and mental presence.

The benefits of mindfulness extend beyond immediate relaxation. Research has shown that regular mindfulness practice can lead to significant improvements in mental health. It has been associated with reductions in stress, anxiety, and depression. Mindfulness helps to cultivate emotional resilience by promoting greater awareness of one's emotional states and fostering a more balanced response to stressors. This enhanced emotional regulation contributes to overall psychological well-being.

Mindfulness also has notable effects on physical health. By reducing stress and promoting relaxation, mindfulness can lower blood pressure, improve sleep quality, and support immune function. The practice's emphasis on relaxation and body awareness can help alleviate chronic pain and improve overall physical comfort.

Incorporating mindfulness into daily life can be achieved through formal practices such as meditation and informal practices such as mindful eating or walking. Formal practices involve setting aside dedicated time for mindfulness exercises, while informal practices involve bringing mindful awareness to everyday activities.

In summary, mindfulness is a practice centered on focusing attention on the present moment with openness and acceptance. By fostering a non-judgmental awareness of thoughts, emotions, and physical sensations, mindfulness promotes mental and physical well-being. Through its various techniques and benefits, mindfulness offers a powerful tool for enhancing overall quality of life and achieving a deeper sense of balance and peace.

3.1 Defining Mindfulness and Its Origins

Mindfulness is a mental practice centered on maintaining a focused and non-judgmental awareness of the present moment. This concept involves observing one's thoughts, emotions, and sensory experiences without becoming overly attached or reactive to them. By fostering an open and accepting attitude toward current experiences, mindfulness aims to cultivate a deeper understanding of oneself and one's surroundings, leading to improved mental clarity, emotional balance, and overall well-being.

The roots of mindfulness can be traced back to ancient contemplative traditions, particularly within Buddhism. The practice has been an integral part of Buddhist philosophy and meditation for over two millennia. In Buddhism, mindfulness, or "sati" in Pali, is one of the central components of the Eightfold Path, which is a guide to ethical and mental development leading to enlightenment. Mindfulness in this context involves maintaining awareness of the Four Foundations of Mindfulness: the body, sensations, mind, and mental objects. By focusing on these aspects, practitioners aim to gain insight into the nature of suffering and the path to liberation.

The concept of mindfulness is not confined to Buddhism; it has also been a significant element in other Eastern traditions, such as Hinduism and Taoism. In Hinduism, practices similar to mindfulness are found in various forms of meditation and yoga, where attention is directed towards breath, bodily sensations, and inner states of being. Taoism, with its emphasis on living in harmony with the Tao (the way or path), also incorporates elements of mindfulness through practices that promote awareness and balance in daily life.

In the West, the modern understanding of mindfulness has been significantly shaped by the work of Jon Kabat-Zinn, a pioneer in integrating mindfulness into mainstream medical and psychological practice. In the late 1970s, Kabat-Zinn developed the Mindfulness-Based Stress Reduction (MBSR) program at the University of Massachusetts Medical School. His approach was designed to help individuals cope with stress, pain, and illness through mindfulness meditation and body awareness. Kabat-Zinn's work was instrumental in bringing mindfulness from its Eastern roots into a secular and clinical context, making it accessible to a broader audience.

The influence of mindfulness has since expanded into various domains of health and well-being, including psychology, therapy, and personal development. Mindfulness-Based Cognitive Therapy (MBCT), developed by Zindel Segal, Mark Williams, and John Teasdale, builds on MBSR by combining mindfulness practices with cognitive behavioral techniques. MBCT is effective in preventing relapse in individuals with recurrent depression and addressing various mental health issues.

Defining mindfulness involves understanding its dual role as both a practice and a state of being. As a practice, mindfulness involves engaging in specific techniques, such as meditation or mindful breathing, to develop and strengthen awareness. As a state of being, mindfulness refers to the ongoing quality of awareness and presence that can be cultivated through practice and integrated into everyday life.

In summary, mindfulness is a practice of focused, non-judgmental awareness of the present moment with origins rooted in ancient contemplative traditions, particularly Buddhism. Its modern adaptation in the West, largely influenced by Jon Kabat-Zinn and subsequent developments, has expanded its application to various fields of health and personal growth. Understanding mindfulness involves recognizing both its historical context and its contemporary relevance in promoting mental clarity, emotional well-being, and overall health.

3.2 Key Principles and Practices of Mindfulness

Mindfulness is anchored in several key principles and practices that together foster a deeper connection to the present moment and enhance overall well-being. These principles and practices are designed to cultivate an attitude of openness, acceptance, and non-judgmental awareness, enabling individuals to engage more fully with their experiences and improve their mental and emotional health.

One fundamental principle of mindfulness is present-moment awareness. This involves focusing attention on the current experience rather than getting lost in thoughts about the past or future. By centering attention on what is happening in the here and now—whether it be physical sensations, emotions, or external events—individuals can develop a clearer understanding of their immediate experience. This principle encourages individuals to experience each moment with full engagement, rather than being distracted or preoccupied.

Non-judgmental observation is another core principle of mindfulness. It involves observing thoughts, feelings, and sensations without labeling them as good or bad. Instead of reacting to experiences with aversion or attraction, mindfulness promotes an attitude of curiosity and acceptance. This non-judgmental stance helps individuals to distance themselves from their reactions and develop a more balanced perspective on their internal experiences. By recognizing and accepting experiences as they are, individuals can reduce the influence of negative judgments and improve emotional resilience.

Acceptance is closely related to non-judgmental observation and involves embracing whatever arises in the present moment without resistance. Acceptance in mindfulness means acknowledging thoughts, emotions, and sensations without trying to change or avoid them. This principle supports the idea that resisting or fighting against unpleasant experiences can exacerbate stress and discomfort while accepting them allows for a more fluid and less reactive approach to challenges.

A key practice within mindfulness is mindful breathing. This practice involves paying close attention to the breath and observing its natural rhythm and sensations. By focusing on the breath, individuals create a stable anchor for their awareness, which helps to center the mind and reduce distractions. Mindful breathing is often used as a starting point for mindfulness meditation and can be practiced throughout the day to bring attention back to the present moment.

Body scans are another common mindfulness practice. This technique involves systematically directing attention to different parts of the body, and observing any sensations, tensions, or discomforts. By performing a body scan, individuals can increase awareness of physical sensations and promote relaxation. This practice helps to cultivate a deeper connection between the mind and body and can be particularly beneficial for managing stress and physical tension.

Mindful movement incorporates mindfulness into physical activities such as yoga, Tai Chi, or walking. This practice involves performing movements with focused attention and awareness, integrating the physical aspects of the activity with mental presence. Mindful movement helps to enhance body awareness, improve flexibility, and foster a sense of calm and balance.

In addition to these practices, mindfulness encourages regular practice and patience. Developing mindfulness is an ongoing process that requires consistent effort and time. Regular practice helps to reinforce mindfulness skills and integrate them into daily life, while patience allows individuals to approach the practice without frustration or expectation.

In summary, the key principles of mindfulness include present-moment awareness, non-judgmental observation, and acceptance. The core practices of mindfulness—such as mindful breathing, body scans, and mindful movement—support these principles and help individuals develop a deeper connection to their experiences. By embracing these principles and practices, individuals can enhance their overall well-being, improve emotional resilience, and cultivate a more mindful approach to daily life.

3.3 The Impact of Mindfulness on Mental and Physical Health

Mindfulness, as a practice of focused and non-judgmental awareness of the present moment, has profound effects on both mental and physical health. Its influence extends across a broad spectrum of well-being, offering benefits that encompass emotional balance, stress reduction, and physical vitality.

One of the most significant impacts of mindfulness is its ability to reduce stress. Chronic stress has been linked to numerous health issues, including cardiovascular problems, weakened immune function, and mental health disorders. Mindfulness practices help mitigate stress by promoting relaxation and activating the parasympathetic nervous system, which counteracts the body's stress response. Through techniques such as mindful breathing and body scans, individuals can cultivate a sense of calm and manage stress more effectively. Research has consistently shown that mindfulness reduces cortisol levels, the hormone associated with stress, leading to lower overall stress levels and improved stress resilience.

In terms of mental health, mindfulness has demonstrated substantial benefits for conditions such as anxiety and depression. By fostering a non-judgmental awareness of thoughts and emotions, mindfulness helps individuals develop a more balanced perspective on their experiences. This approach reduces rumination—repetitive and often negative thinking patterns that are common in both anxiety and depression. Mindfulness-Based Cognitive Therapy (MBCT), which combines mindfulness practices with cognitive behavioral techniques, has been shown to prevent relapse in individuals with recurrent depression and improve symptoms of anxiety. The practice promotes emotional regulation and enhances the ability to respond to challenging situations with greater equanimity.

Mindfulness also plays a crucial role in enhancing overall emotional well-being. By increasing self-awareness and encouraging acceptance, mindfulness helps individuals build a more positive relationship with their emotions. This greater awareness allows individuals to identify and address negative emotional patterns and cultivate a more positive outlook on life. The practice of mindfulness encourages self-compassion and reduces self-criticism, contributing to improved self-esteem and emotional resilience.

On a physical level, mindfulness contributes to better health outcomes by improving physiological processes and promoting overall well-being. Studies have shown that mindfulness practices can lower blood pressure, improve heart rate variability, and enhance immune function. By reducing stress and promoting relaxation, mindfulness supports cardiovascular health and helps mitigate the negative effects of chronic stress on the body. Additionally, mindfulness has been associated with improved sleep quality, which is crucial for physical recovery and overall health. Techniques such as mindful breathing and body scans can aid in overcoming insomnia and promoting restorative sleep.

Mindfulness also aids in pain management and can improve the quality of life for individuals experiencing chronic pain. By shifting the focus away from the discomfort and fostering a more accepting and non-reactive approach to pain, mindfulness helps individuals manage their pain more effectively. Mindfulness-Based Stress Reduction (MBSR) programs have been shown to reduce the perception of pain and improve coping strategies, contributing to a better overall experience of chronic pain conditions.

Furthermore, mindfulness promotes healthier lifestyle choices and behaviors. Individuals who practice mindfulness are more likely to engage in behaviors that support their well-being, such as regular physical activity, healthy eating, and adequate self-care. This holistic approach to health emphasizes the integration of mindfulness into daily life, leading to more mindful decision-making and improved overall health.

In summary, mindfulness has a significant impact on both mental and physical health. By reducing stress, improving emotional regulation, and enhancing overall well-being, mindfulness contributes to a more balanced and healthy life. Its benefits extend to physical health as well, including better cardiovascular function, improved immune response, and effective pain management. Through its holistic approach, mindfulness supports comprehensive health and well-being, fostering a greater sense of balance and vitality.

Chapter 4: Integrating Massage and Mindfulness

Integrating massage therapy with mindfulness practices creates a powerful synergy that enhances both physical relaxation and mental clarity. This combined approach leverages the strengths of each discipline to promote holistic well-being, addressing both the body and mind cohesively.

Massage therapy and mindfulness both emphasize the importance of being present and attentive to the current moment. When these practices are integrated, they amplify the benefits of each other, leading to a deeper state of relaxation and increased awareness. During a massage, the physical touch and manipulation of muscles help release tension and promote a sense of calm. When combined with mindfulness, this process becomes more profound, as individuals are encouraged to stay fully present with the sensations of the massage. This heightened awareness allows for a more immersive experience, leading to greater relaxation and a deeper connection with the body.

The practice of mindful massage involves bringing attention to the physical sensations experienced during the massage. This means focusing on the feeling of the therapist's hands, the texture of the skin, and the release of tension in the muscles. By maintaining a mindful awareness throughout the massage, individuals can enhance their sensory experience and deepen their relaxation. This approach also helps individuals to be more attuned to their body's needs and responses, which can improve the effectiveness of the massage.

Mindfulness techniques can also be incorporated into the massage process to further enhance the benefits. For example, mindful breathing exercises can be used to help individuals stay centered and present during the massage. By focusing on slow, deep breaths, individuals can calm their nervous system and support the relaxation response. This practice not only enhances the physical benefits of the massage but also helps to reduce mental stress and anxiety.

Another way to integrate mindfulness with massage is through guided imagery or visualization. During the massage, individuals can be guided to visualize a peaceful and calming environment, such as a serene beach or a tranquil forest. This visualization can enhance the relaxation experience and provide a mental escape from daily stressors. By combining the physical sensations of the massage with a calming mental image, individuals can achieve a deeper state of relaxation and mental clarity.

In addition to enhancing the massage experience, integrating mindfulness into daily life can support long-term well-being. Mindfulness practices, such as meditation and mindful movement, can be used to complement the benefits of regular massage therapy. By cultivating a mindful attitude in everyday activities, individuals can maintain a greater sense of balance and reduce stress, which can enhance the overall effectiveness of massage therapy.

The integration of massage and mindfulness also supports emotional and psychological well-being. The combination of physical touch and mindful awareness helps to address both physical tension and emotional stress, fostering a holistic sense of well-being. This integrated approach encourages individuals to explore and address emotional blockages that may be stored in the body, leading to greater emotional release and healing.

In summary, integrating massage therapy with mindfulness creates a synergistic approach that enhances both physical and mental well-being. By combining the physical relaxation of massage with the present-moment awareness of mindfulness, individuals can achieve a deeper state of relaxation, improve body awareness, and support overall health. This integrated approach not only enhances the immediate benefits of each practice but also contributes to long-term well-being by fostering a balanced and mindful approach to life.

4.1 How to Combine Massage and Mindfulness for Enhanced Well-Being

Combining massage therapy with mindfulness can significantly enhance overall well-being by addressing both physical relaxation and mental clarity. This integration leverages the strengths of each practice to create a holistic approach that promotes deeper relaxation, improved body awareness, and emotional balance. To effectively combine massage and mindfulness, several strategies can be employed to maximize the benefits of each practice.

The first step in combining massage and mindfulness is to establish a mindful approach during the massage session. This involves cultivating a heightened awareness of the present moment and focusing on the sensations experienced during the massage. As the therapist works on different areas of the body, individuals are encouraged to pay close attention to the physical sensations, such as the pressure of the therapist's hands, the warmth of the oil, and the release of muscle tension. By maintaining this mindful focus, individuals can deepen their relaxation and fully engage with the massage experience.

Incorporating mindful breathing into the massage session can further enhance the benefits. Mindful breathing involves focusing on the rhythm and sensation of each breath, helping to calm the nervous system and support the relaxation response. Before or during the massage, individuals can practice deep, slow breathing to create a calming effect. This practice helps to reduce stress and anxiety, allowing the body to relax more fully and the mind to remain present. Coordinating breath with the rhythm of the massage can also amplify the sense of relaxation and connection.

Another effective method of integrating mindfulness into the massage experience is through guided imagery or visualization. This technique involves using the imagination to create a mental picture of a peaceful and calming environment. During the massage, individuals can be guided to visualize a serene setting, such as a quiet beach or a lush forest. This visualization helps to enhance the relaxation experience by providing a mental escape from everyday stressors. The combination of physical touch and a calming mental image can lead to a deeper state of relaxation and mental clarity.

In addition to mindfulness practices during the massage, incorporating mindfulness into daily life can support long-term well-being and complement the benefits of massage therapy. Regular mindfulness practices, such as meditation or mindful movement, can help individuals maintain a greater sense of balance and reduce stress outside of the massage session. By developing a consistent mindfulness practice, individuals can enhance their overall emotional resilience and improve their ability to manage stress, which in turn can make the effects of massage therapy more enduring.

Creating a mindful environment for the massage session is also important. This involves setting up a tranquil and calming space where individuals can relax without distractions. Elements such as soft lighting, soothing music, and a comfortable temperature contribute to a peaceful atmosphere that supports mindfulness. Ensuring that the environment is conducive to relaxation can enhance the overall experience and help individuals remain focused on the present moment.

In summary, combining massage therapy with mindfulness can lead to enhanced well-being by integrating the physical relaxation of massage with the mental clarity of mindfulness. By cultivating mindful awareness during the massage, incorporating mindful breathing and guided imagery, and creating a tranquil environment, individuals can achieve a deeper level of relaxation and emotional balance. Integrating mindfulness into daily life further supports long-term well-being and enhances the overall effectiveness of massage therapy. This holistic approach fosters a greater sense of connection between the body and mind, contributing to overall health and vitality.

4.2 Techniques for Incorporating Mindfulness into Massage Sessions

Incorporating mindfulness into massage sessions can profoundly enhance the overall therapeutic experience by fostering a deeper connection between the mind and body. This integration involves using specific techniques to cultivate a heightened sense of awareness, relaxation, and presence throughout the massage. Here are some effective methods to achieve this integration:

One key technique is mindful breathing. Before beginning the massage, both the therapist and the client can engage in deep, intentional breathing exercises. The client is encouraged to focus on their breath, inhaling deeply through the nose and exhaling slowly through the mouth. This practice helps to center the mind, calm the nervous system, and prepare the body for relaxation. During the massage, the therapist can guide the client to maintain this mindful breathing rhythm, which enhances the relaxation response and helps to keep the client present with the sensations of the massage.

Body scan awareness is another technique that can be effectively integrated into a massage session. This involves guiding the client to mentally scan their body, paying attention to various areas of tension or discomfort. The therapist can encourage the client to bring their awareness to specific areas as they work on them, helping them to notice subtle sensations and shifts in tension. By focusing on these areas with a sense of curiosity and acceptance, clients can achieve a deeper level of relaxation and release.

Mindful touch is a technique that involves the therapist being fully present and attentive to the act of touching and manipulating the client's body. This means applying a gentle and deliberate touch and paying close attention to the client's feedback and physical responses. The therapist's mindfulness can influence the quality of the massage, creating a more attuned and responsive therapeutic experience. This mindful approach to touch helps to foster a deeper connection between the therapist and client, enhancing the overall effectiveness of the massage.

Guided imagery can also be used during a massage to enhance mindfulness. The therapist may guide the client through a visualization exercise, inviting them to imagine a serene and calming environment. This could be a peaceful beach, a quiet forest, or any other tranquil setting that resonates with the client. By focusing on this mental image, clients can further relax and detach from everyday stressors, enriching the massage experience and promoting a greater sense of mental clarity.

Integrating affirmations into the massage can also be beneficial. The therapist can offer positive affirmations or supportive words throughout the session, encouraging the client to maintain a positive and accepting attitude. These affirmations can help reinforce the client's focus on the present moment and foster a deeper sense of relaxation and well-being.

Finally, creating a mindful environment is crucial for integrating mindfulness into the massage session. The therapist should ensure that the space is calm and conducive to relaxation, with elements such as soft lighting, soothing music, and a comfortable temperature. This mindful setup helps to create an atmosphere that supports the client's ability to remain present and fully engaged in the massage.

In summary, incorporating mindfulness into massage sessions involves using techniques such as mindful breathing, body scan awareness, mindful touch, guided imagery, and affirmations to enhance the therapeutic experience. By cultivating a mindful approach, both the therapist and the client can achieve a deeper level of relaxation, presence, and connection. Creating a tranquil environment further supports this integration, leading to a more effective and holistic massage experience that promotes overall well-being.

4.3 Case Studies: Success Stories of Integrating Both Practices

Integrating massage therapy with mindfulness has proven to be a transformative approach for many individuals seeking to enhance their physical and mental well-being. Several case studies highlight the profound benefits that arise from combining these practices, showcasing how this integration can address a variety of health concerns and improve overall quality of life.

One compelling case is that of Sarah, a 42-year-old professional who had been experiencing chronic stress and anxiety. Despite trying various stress management techniques, Sarah found little relief until she began combining massage therapy with mindfulness practices. Her massage therapist incorporated mindful breathing and body scan techniques into each session, guiding Sarah to focus on her breath and body sensations. This approach helped Sarah to become more aware of the physical manifestations of her stress and allowed her to release accumulated tension more effectively. Over time, Sarah reported significant reductions in her anxiety levels and an improved sense of overall well-being. She also noticed enhanced resilience in handling daily stressors and a greater ability to remain present and engaged in her work and personal life.

Another success story involves John, a 56-year-old individual suffering from chronic lower back pain. Traditional treatments had provided only temporary relief, so John sought an alternative approach. His massage therapist integrated mindfulness into the sessions by incorporating guided imagery and mindful touch techniques. During the massages, John was guided to visualize a serene landscape while focusing on the sensations in his lower back. This combination of physical touch and mental relaxation led to a notable decrease in pain and discomfort. John found that the mindfulness practices not only helped alleviate his back pain but also contributed to a more positive outlook on his condition. The enhanced mind-body connection allowed him to manage his pain more effectively and improved his overall quality of life.

A third case study features Emily, a 30-year-old with a history of insomnia and frequent emotional stress. Her insomnia was exacerbated by a high-stress job and difficulty relaxing at night. Emily decided to explore the integration of massage and mindfulness as a potential solution. Her therapist incorporated mindful breathing exercises and affirmations into the massage sessions. By focusing on calming breathwork and positive affirmations, Emily was able to achieve a deeper state of relaxation during and after the massages. Over several weeks, she experienced significant improvements in sleep quality and a reduction in nighttime anxiety. The combination of physical relaxation from the massage and mental calmness from mindfulness practices helped her develop healthier sleep patterns and a more balanced emotional state.

A final case study involves Mark, a 45-year-old recovering from a traumatic injury. Mark faced challenges with both physical pain and emotional trauma, which hindered his recovery. His treatment plan included combining massage therapy with mindfulness practices. The therapist used body scan techniques to help Mark become more aware of areas of tension and pain while integrating mindfulness to address emotional trauma. Through guided imagery and mindful touch, Mark was able to process and release emotional blockages associated with his injury. This holistic approach contributed to a more comprehensive recovery process, leading to improvements in both physical comfort and emotional well-being.

These case studies illustrate the powerful impact of integrating massage therapy with mindfulness. By addressing both physical and mental aspects of health, individuals can experience profound benefits, including reduced stress, pain relief, improved sleep, and enhanced overall well-being. The success stories demonstrate how the synergy between these practices can create a more effective and holistic approach to health and recovery.

Chapter 5: Developing a Holistic Wellness Routine

Creating a holistic wellness routine involves integrating practices that support physical health, mental clarity, and emotional balance into daily life. Such a routine is designed to address the interconnected nature of well-being, promoting overall health through a balanced approach that considers the body, mind, and spirit. Developing an effective holistic wellness routine requires thoughtful planning and consistency, with an emphasis on practices that harmonize and complement each other.

To begin developing a holistic wellness routine, it is essential to start with self-assessment. Understanding individual needs and goals is crucial for creating a personalized routine that addresses specific health concerns and preferences. This involves reflecting on areas such as physical fitness, mental health, stress levels, and lifestyle habits. By identifying personal strengths and areas for improvement, individuals can tailor their routines to meet their unique needs and aspirations.

A core component of a holistic wellness routine is physical activity. Regular exercise is fundamental to maintaining physical health and vitality. Incorporating a variety of activities, such as cardiovascular exercises, strength training, and flexibility workouts, can provide comprehensive benefits. Activities like walking, jogging, swimming, or yoga can enhance cardiovascular health, build muscle strength, and improve flexibility. The key is to choose activities that are enjoyable and sustainable, as consistency is vital for long-term success.

In addition to physical exercise, nutrition plays a significant role in overall wellness. A balanced diet that includes a variety of whole foods, such as fruits, vegetables, lean proteins, and whole grains, supports optimal health and energy levels. It is also important to stay hydrated by drinking plenty of water throughout the day. Nutritional choices should focus on providing the body with essential nutrients and avoiding excessive consumption of processed foods, sugars, and unhealthy fats.

Mindfulness and stress management are essential aspects of a holistic wellness routine. Incorporating mindfulness practices, such as meditation, deep breathing exercises, and mindful movement, can help manage stress and promote mental clarity. Regular mindfulness practice helps individuals stay present, reduce anxiety, and improve emotional regulation. Techniques like progressive muscle relaxation or guided imagery can also enhance relaxation and contribute to overall well-being.

Sleep is another crucial element of a holistic wellness routine. Quality sleep is essential for physical recovery, cognitive function, and emotional balance. Establishing a consistent sleep schedule, creating a restful sleep environment, and practicing good sleep hygiene can improve sleep quality. This includes avoiding screens before bedtime, maintaining a comfortable sleep environment, and engaging in relaxing pre-sleep rituals, such as reading or gentle stretching.

Self-care practices, including activities that promote relaxation and personal enjoyment, should be integrated into the routine. Activities such as reading, hobbies, spending time in nature, or engaging in creative pursuits contribute to emotional well-being and personal fulfillment. Regular self-care helps to recharge and rejuvenate, providing a necessary balance to the demands of daily life.

Social connections and relationships also play a vital role in holistic wellness. Building and maintaining positive relationships with family, friends, and community can provide emotional support, reduce feelings of isolation, and enhance overall happiness. Engaging in social activities and fostering meaningful connections contribute to a sense of belonging and well-being.

Lastly, it is important to evaluate and adjust the routine regularly. As life circumstances and personal needs evolve, the wellness routine may require adjustments to remain effective. Regularly assessing progress and making necessary changes ensures that the routine continues to support well-being and meets evolving goals.

In summary, developing a holistic wellness routine involves integrating physical activity, balanced nutrition, mindfulness practices, quality sleep, self-care, and social connections into daily life. By addressing these interconnected aspects of well-being and maintaining consistency, individuals can achieve a balanced and fulfilling lifestyle that supports overall health and happiness.

5.1 Creating a Balanced Routine with Massage and Mindfulness

Integrating massage therapy and mindfulness into a balanced wellness routine offers a comprehensive approach to enhancing physical and mental health. Both practices complement each other by addressing relaxation, stress management, and overall well-being, and incorporating them into a routine requires thoughtful planning and consistency.

To create a balanced routine that incorporates both massage and mindfulness, start by establishing regular massage sessions. Regular massage therapy is beneficial for relieving muscle tension, reducing stress, and promoting relaxation. Depending on individual needs and preferences, this might involve scheduling sessions weekly, biweekly, or monthly. The key is to find a frequency that aligns with personal goals and fits comfortably into one's schedule. Consistency in receiving massages allows the body to continuously benefit from the therapeutic effects, supporting long-term well-being.

Mindfulness practices should be incorporated daily to complement the benefits of massage therapy. These practices can include meditation, mindful breathing, and mindful movement. Starting each day with a brief mindfulness session, such as a 10-minute meditation or deep breathing exercise, sets a positive tone and fosters mental clarity. This daily practice helps manage stress and cultivates a greater sense of present-moment awareness, which can enhance the benefits received from massage therapy.

Integrating mindfulness into the massage experience itself can further enhance its effectiveness. During massage sessions, focus on mindful awareness by paying close attention to the physical sensations and the process of relaxation. This can involve being fully present with the touch, pressure, and movement of the massage, as well as tuning into any areas of tension or discomfort. Mindful awareness during the massage helps deepen the relaxation response and allows individuals to connect more profoundly with their body's needs.

Incorporating mindful techniques into everyday activities can also support a balanced routine. For example, practice mindful eating by savoring each bite and paying attention to the flavors, textures, and sensations of the food. This approach not only enhances the enjoyment of meals but also supports healthier eating habits. Additionally, incorporating mindfulness into daily tasks, such as walking or even during work breaks, can help maintain a sense of calm and focus throughout the day.

Self-care practices that align with massage and mindfulness can further contribute to a balanced routine. Activities such as taking relaxing baths, engaging in gentle stretching exercises, or practicing yoga can enhance the overall sense of relaxation and well-being. These practices complement the benefits of massage and mindfulness by providing additional opportunities for physical and mental rejuvenation.

To ensure the routine remains balanced and effective, it is important to evaluate and adjust it regularly. Assessing how well the integration of massage and mindfulness is meeting personal goals and needs allows for adjustments as necessary. This might involve altering the frequency of massage sessions, experimenting with different mindfulness techniques, or incorporating new self-care activities. Flexibility and responsiveness to changing needs help maintain a routine that continues to support overall well-being.

In summary, creating a balanced routine with massage and mindfulness involves integrating regular massage sessions with daily mindfulness practices. By incorporating mindful awareness during massages, applying mindfulness techniques to everyday activities, and engaging in complementary self-care practices, individuals can achieve a comprehensive approach to physical and mental well-being. Regular evaluation and adjustment of the routine ensure it remains aligned with personal needs and continues to promote overall health and happiness.

5.2 Daily and Weekly Practices for Optimal Health

Maintaining optimal health requires a balanced combination of daily and weekly practices that support physical, mental, and emotional well-being. By incorporating a variety of habits into your routine, you can foster a holistic approach to health that enhances overall quality of life. These practices should be tailored to individual needs and preferences, ensuring they are both effective and sustainable.

Daily practices form the foundation of a healthy routine and should be designed to address key areas of well-being. Physical activity is a crucial daily practice for maintaining cardiovascular health, muscle strength, and flexibility. Aim for at least 30 minutes of moderate exercise each day, such as brisk walking, jogging, or cycling. Incorporating a mix of activities that include cardiovascular, strength, and flexibility exercises helps to ensure comprehensive fitness. For those with busy schedules, breaking the exercise into shorter segments throughout the day can also be effective.

Mindfulness and relaxation techniques should be incorporated into your daily routine to support mental clarity and stress management. Practicing mindfulness through meditation or deep breathing exercises for just 10 to 15 minutes each day can help reduce stress, improve focus, and enhance emotional resilience. Engaging in mindful activities, such as mindful eating or mindful walking, can also promote a sense of calm and present-moment awareness throughout the day.

Healthy eating is another essential daily practice. Consuming a balanced diet that includes a variety of whole foods—such as fruits, vegetables, lean proteins, and whole grains—supports overall health and provides the body with essential nutrients. Pay attention to portion sizes and aim to eat meals at regular intervals to maintain stable energy levels. Staying hydrated by drinking adequate amounts of water is also important for bodily functions and overall well-being.

Quality sleep should be prioritized daily to ensure physical and mental recovery. Establish a consistent sleep schedule by going to bed and waking up at the same time each day. Create a restful sleep environment by keeping the room dark, cool, and quiet. Engaging in relaxing pre-sleep rituals, such as reading or gentle stretching, can help signal to the body that it's time to wind down.

Weekly practices complement daily routines by providing additional opportunities for holistic health. Massage therapy, for example, can be integrated on a weekly or biweekly basis to relieve muscle tension, enhance relaxation, and promote overall well-being. Regular massages help to release accumulated stress and improve circulation, supporting both physical and mental health.

Self-care activities should be scheduled weekly to recharge and rejuvenate. This might include setting aside time for hobbies, engaging in creative pursuits, or enjoying activities that bring joy and relaxation. These self-care practices contribute to emotional well-being and help balance the demands of daily life.

Social connections and relationships also play a significant role in well-being. Make an effort to connect with family and friends every week, whether through social gatherings, phone calls, or other forms of communication. Positive social interactions provide emotional support, reduce feelings of isolation, and enhance overall happiness.

Weekly reflection is an important practice for maintaining a balanced routine. Take time to assess your progress, evaluate what's working well, and identify any areas that may need adjustment. Reflecting on your goals and experiences helps to ensure that your practices remain aligned with your well-being objectives and allows for necessary adjustments to maintain a healthy balance.

In summary, optimizing health involves a combination of daily and weekly practices that support physical, mental, and emotional well-being. Daily habits such as regular exercise, mindfulness, healthy eating, and quality sleep lay the foundation for overall health, while weekly practices like massage therapy, self-care, social connections, and reflection provide additional support and enhancement. By integrating these practices into your routine, you can achieve a comprehensive approach to well-being that promotes a healthier, more balanced life.

5.3 Setting and Achieving Wellness Goals

Setting and achieving wellness goals is a crucial component of maintaining and enhancing overall health. Effective goal-setting not only provides direction and motivation but also helps individuals create a structured approach to improving their well-being. To successfully set and achieve wellness goals, it is important to follow a systematic process that includes defining clear objectives, creating actionable plans, and maintaining motivation throughout the journey.

The first step in setting wellness goals is to establish clear and specific objectives. Wellness goals should be well-defined and tailored to individual needs and aspirations. This involves reflecting on areas of improvement, such as physical fitness, mental health, nutrition, or stress management. For instance, a clear goal might be to increase physical activity levels by committing to exercise for 30 minutes a day, five days a week. Specificity helps in creating a concrete plan and provides a benchmark against which progress can be measured.

Once objectives are defined, it is important to create actionable plans. This involves breaking down larger goals into smaller, manageable steps. For example, if the goal is to improve dietary habits, the plan might include steps such as meal planning, incorporating more fruits and vegetables into daily meals, and reducing the intake of processed foods. Each step should be realistic and achievable, providing a clear path towards the overall goal. Creating a schedule or timeline for these steps helps in maintaining focus and ensures consistent progress.

To enhance the likelihood of success, it is beneficial to establish measurable milestones. These milestones act as checkpoints that allow individuals to monitor their progress and make adjustments as needed. For example, if the goal is to lose weight, milestones might include tracking weight loss over weeks or months and celebrating small achievements along the way. Measuring progress helps in maintaining motivation and provides a sense of accomplishment as goals are met.

Maintaining motivation is a key aspect of achieving wellness goals. This can be supported through various strategies, such as setting up a reward system for reaching milestones, seeking support from friends or a wellness coach, and regularly reviewing and adjusting goals as needed.

Staying connected to the reasons for setting the goal and visualizing the benefits of achieving it can also help sustain motivation. Additionally, incorporating goal-setting into daily or weekly routines ensures that wellness remains a priority and reinforces commitment.

Overcoming obstacles is an inevitable part of the goal-setting process. Challenges such as lack of time, unexpected events, or setbacks can arise, potentially hindering progress. It is important to anticipate potential obstacles and develop strategies for addressing them. This might involve creating a contingency plan, adjusting goals to be more realistic, or seeking support when needed. Flexibility and resilience are crucial in navigating these challenges and maintaining progress toward wellness goals.

Regular reflection and reassessment are essential for successful goal achievement. Periodically reviewing progress allows individuals to evaluate what is working well and what may need adjustment. This reflection helps in identifying any changes in needs or priorities and provides an opportunity to refine goals and plans. Adjusting goals as necessary ensures that they remain relevant and achievable, supporting ongoing progress and well-being.

In summary, setting and achieving wellness goals involves defining clear objectives, creating actionable plans, establishing measurable milestones, and maintaining motivation. By anticipating obstacles, remaining flexible, and regularly reflecting on progress, individuals can successfully reach their wellness goals and enhance their overall health. This structured approach fosters a proactive mindset and supports long-term well-being, leading to a more balanced and fulfilling life.

Chapter 6: Mindfulness Techniques for Enhancing Massage

Integrating mindfulness techniques into massage therapy can profoundly enhance the therapeutic experience by deepening relaxation, improving body awareness, and fostering a stronger mind-body connection. These techniques help clients fully engage with the massage, making the experience more effective and restorative. By combining the physical benefits of massage with the mental clarity of mindfulness, practitioners and clients alike can achieve a more holistic approach to wellness.

One of the primary mindfulness techniques for enhancing massage is mindful breathing. This practice involves focusing attention on the breath and observing each inhalation and exhalation without judgment. Before or during a massage session, clients can be guided to take slow, deep breaths, which helps to calm the nervous system and prepare the body for relaxation. Mindful breathing can enhance the body's ability to release tension and increase the overall effectiveness of the massage. By synchronizing breath with the rhythm of the massage, clients can achieve a deeper state of relaxation and awareness.

Body scan awareness is another powerful mindfulness technique that can be integrated into massage sessions. This technique involves guiding clients to mentally scan their bodies, paying attention to areas of tension or discomfort. During the massage, clients can be encouraged to focus on specific areas as they are being worked on, helping them to become more aware of their physical sensations and the release of tension. This heightened awareness allows clients to connect more deeply with their bodies and enhances the therapeutic effects of the massage.

Mindful touch involves both the therapist and client being fully present during the massage. For therapists, this means applying a deliberate and attentive touch and being sensitive to the client's feedback and physical responses. For clients, it involves focusing on the sensations of touch, pressure, and movement during the massage. Mindful touch helps to create a more attuned and responsive therapeutic experience, enhancing relaxation and improving the overall effectiveness of the massage.

Incorporating guided imagery into the massage session can also enhance mindfulness. This technique involves guiding clients to visualize a serene and calming environment, such as a peaceful beach or a tranquil forest. This mental imagery helps clients to relax more deeply and escape from everyday stressors. The combination of physical touch and a calming mental image can create a more immersive and restorative experience, further amplifying the benefits of the massage.

Affirmations and positive suggestions can be used during the massage to reinforce mindfulness and relaxation. Therapists can offer gentle, supportive affirmations or phrases that encourage clients to let go of stress and embrace a sense of calm. These positive suggestions help to create a more soothing environment and can enhance the client's overall experience by promoting a positive and relaxed state of mind.

Creating a mindful environment is also essential for enhancing the massage experience. This involves setting up a calming atmosphere with elements such as soft lighting, soothing music, and a comfortable temperature. A tranquil environment supports mindfulness by helping clients focus on the present moment and fully engage with the massage experience.

In summary, integrating mindfulness techniques into massage therapy involves practices such as mindful breathing, body scan awareness, mindful touch, guided imagery, and positive affirmations. By incorporating these techniques, both therapists and clients can achieve a deeper level of relaxation, awareness, and therapeutic benefit. Creating a mindful environment further enhances the overall experience, leading to a more effective and restorative massage that supports holistic well-being.

6.1 Mindfulness Practices to Prepare for a Massage Session

Preparing for a massage session with mindfulness practices can significantly enhance the effectiveness of the therapy by setting the stage for deep relaxation and optimal benefits. Mindfulness practices help clients arrive at the session with a calm and focused mind, creating a conducive environment for therapeutic work. By integrating mindfulness into the preparation process, clients can maximize the therapeutic potential of the massage and foster a more profound sense of well-being.

The first mindfulness practice to consider is mindful breathing. Before the massage session begins, clients can engage in deep, intentional breathing exercises to center themselves and calm their nervous system. This practice involves sitting comfortably and focusing on the natural rhythm of the breath. By taking slow, deep breaths in through the nose and out through the mouth, clients can reduce stress and anxiety, creating a more relaxed state. This initial calmness helps to prepare the body for the massage, allowing for a more effective release of tension.

Body scan awareness is another valuable mindfulness practice to incorporate before a massage. This technique involves mentally scanning the body from head to toe, paying attention to areas of tension, discomfort, or stress. Clients can take a few moments to observe and acknowledge these sensations without judgment. By identifying areas of physical discomfort, clients can communicate these concerns to the therapist, ensuring that the massage is tailored to address specific needs. Additionally, this practice helps clients to become more aware of their bodies, promoting a deeper connection and enhancing the overall massage experience.

Setting intentions is a mindfulness practice that can further enhance the massage session. Before arriving at the session, clients can take a moment to reflect on what they hope to achieve from the massage. This might include intentions such as reducing stress, alleviating muscle tension, or improving overall relaxation. By setting clear intentions, clients can focus their mental energy on their goals for the session, which can help to guide the therapist's approach and make the session more purposeful. This intentional focus also supports a more mindful and engaged experience during the massage.

Visualization techniques can also be useful in preparing for a massage. Clients can imagine a peaceful and calming environment, such as a serene beach or a tranquil forest, and mentally transport themselves to this setting. This visualization helps to create a sense of relaxation and mental escape, which can enhance the body's response to the massage. By focusing on a calming mental image, clients can shift their attention away from everyday stressors and immerse themselves in a state of tranquility.

In addition to these practices, clients should ensure that they arrive at the massage session with a comfortable and relaxed mindset. This involves allowing enough time to get to the session without feeling rushed and ensuring that they are mentally prepared to fully engage with the experience. Arriving with a relaxed mindset helps clients to be more receptive to the therapeutic effects of the massage and supports a more effective and enjoyable session.

Communicating openly with the therapist is also an important aspect of preparation. Clients should feel comfortable discussing any specific areas of concern, preferences, or medical conditions with the therapist. This open communication helps the therapist tailor the massage to meet individual needs and ensures that the session addresses the client's goals and preferences.

In summary, mindfulness practices such as mindful breathing, body scan awareness, setting intentions, and visualization techniques can significantly enhance the preparation for a massage session. By incorporating these practices, clients can create a state of relaxation and mental clarity that supports the effectiveness of the massage and fosters a more profound sense of well-being.

6.2 Using Breathwork and Meditation to Enhance the Massage Experience

Integrating breathwork and meditation into the massage experience can profoundly enhance its benefits, fostering deeper relaxation and a stronger mind-body connection. Both practices support the therapeutic process by promoting calmness, increasing body awareness, and helping clients fully engage with the massage. By incorporating these techniques, individuals can experience a more holistic and restorative massage.

Breathwork is a foundational practice that can significantly enhance the massage experience. Deep, intentional breathing helps to activate the parasympathetic nervous system, which is responsible for the body's rest-and-digest responses. Before the massage begins, clients can engage in a series of deep breaths, inhaling slowly through the nose and exhaling gently through the mouth. This breathwork helps to calm the nervous system, lower stress levels, and prepare the body for relaxation. During the massage, maintaining a focus on the breath can further deepen relaxation. Clients can coordinate their breathing with the rhythm of the massage, inhaling as the therapist applies pressure and exhaling as the pressure is released. This synchrony between breath and touch enhances the overall experience, allowing for a more profound sense of release and relaxation.

Meditation before and during the massage can also play a crucial role in enhancing the therapeutic effects. Pre-massage meditation involves setting aside a few minutes to practice mindfulness or guided meditation. This practice helps to clear the mind, reduce anxiety, and shift focus away from daily stressors. Clients might use meditation techniques such as focusing on a mantra or visualizing a peaceful scene to enter a state of calm. This mental preparation sets a tranquil tone for the massage, making it easier to achieve a deeper level of relaxation.

During the massage, meditation techniques can be integrated to maintain focus and enhance the experience. One approach is to practice body scan meditation, where clients mentally observe sensations in different parts of their body. This practice encourages a heightened awareness of physical sensations and allows clients to notice and appreciate the therapeutic effects of the massage more fully. By remaining mindful of how different areas of the body respond to touch and pressure, clients can experience a greater sense of connection with the massage process.

Guided imagery is another meditation technique that can enhance the massage experience. Clients can use guided imagery to mentally transport themselves to a serene and calming environment, such as a quiet beach or a peaceful forest. This mental visualization can complement the physical sensations of the massage, creating a more immersive and restorative experience. By focusing on soothing imagery, clients can further relax and escape from everyday stress, enhancing the overall therapeutic benefits of the session.

Breath awareness during the massage involves paying close attention to the natural rhythm of the breath and using it as a tool for relaxation. Clients can practice observing their breath without altering it, simply noting the sensations of inhalation and exhalation. This awareness helps to keep the mind focused and calm, reducing distractions and promoting a deeper state of relaxation. By incorporating breath awareness into the massage, clients can achieve a more mindful and present experience.

Incorporating breathwork and meditation into the massage experience supports a more comprehensive approach to relaxation and well-being. Breathwork helps to calm the nervous system and synchronize with the massage rhythm, while meditation techniques such as body scan, guided imagery, and breath awareness enhance mental focus and relaxation. By integrating these practices, clients can achieve a more profound and restorative massage experience, fostering a deeper sense of calm and connection.

6.3 Post-Massage Mindfulness: Continuing the Benefits

Post-massage mindfulness is essential for extending the benefits of the massage experience and ensuring that the therapeutic effects are fully integrated into daily life. Mindfulness practices following a massage session help maintain a state of relaxation, deepen body awareness, and support overall well-being. By incorporating mindful practices into the post-massage period, individuals can enhance the benefits of the massage and foster a more enduring sense of calm and balance.

Immediately after the massage, taking a few moments for mindful reflection helps to solidify the sense of relaxation and awareness achieved during the session. Clients can sit quietly, focusing on their breath and the sensations in their bodies. This period of reflection allows them to notice any residual effects of the massage, such as reduced muscle tension or increased relaxation, and appreciate the therapeutic work that has been done. Mindful reflection helps to anchor the relaxation achieved during the massage and encourages a continued state of calm.

Gentle movement and stretching can also be beneficial post-massage. Engaging in gentle, mindful stretching exercises allows the body to integrate the benefits of the massage and maintain flexibility. Simple stretches, such as reaching for the sky or gently bending side to side, can help release any remaining tension and keep the body relaxed. Performing these stretches mindfully, paying attention to how the body feels and moves, supports a smooth transition from the massage session to daily activities.

To continue the benefits of massage, incorporating mindful hydration and nutrition into the post-massage routine is important. Drinking water helps to flush out toxins released during the massage and supports overall hydration. Clients should also consider consuming a balanced meal or snack that includes hydrating foods and nutrients that aid in muscle recovery. Eating mindfully, by savoring each bite and paying attention to the body's hunger and fullness cues, reinforces the sense of well-being achieved through the massage.

Mindful breathing exercises can be used to maintain the relaxation achieved during the massage. Taking a few minutes to engage in deep, intentional breathing helps to calm the mind and body and reinforces the therapeutic effects of the session. Breathing deeply and slowly, focusing on each inhale and exhale, helps to sustain a state of relaxation and manage any lingering stress.

Incorporating mindfulness into daily activities following a massage session extends the benefits of the therapy throughout the day. Being present and mindful during routine activities—such as walking, working, or engaging in conversations—helps to maintain the calm and relaxation achieved during the massage. This mindfulness practice promotes a more balanced and centered approach to daily life, reducing stress and enhancing overall well-being.

Self-care practices following a massage can further support the integration of its benefits. Engaging in activities that promote relaxation and personal enjoyment, such as taking a warm bath, listening to calming music, or practicing gentle yoga, helps to reinforce the sense of calm and relaxation. These self-care practices complement the effects of the massage and contribute to ongoing well-being.

Finally, journaling or noting reflections about the massage experience can help clients process and integrate the benefits. Writing about feelings, observations, and any changes in physical or emotional states provides insight and reinforces the positive effects of the massage. This reflective practice helps clients remain connected to the benefits of the massage and supports continued mindfulness and well-being.

In summary, post-massage mindfulness practices, such as mindful reflection, gentle movement, hydration, mindful breathing, and self-care, are crucial for extending the benefits of the massage. By incorporating these practices into the post-massage routine, individuals can maintain relaxation, deepen body awareness, and support overall well-being, ensuring that the therapeutic effects of the massage continue to enhance daily life.

Chapter 7: Addressing Common Health Concerns with Massage and Mindfulness

Massage and mindfulness are powerful tools that can address a wide range of common health concerns, offering relief and improving overall well-being. By integrating these practices into daily life, individuals can manage symptoms, enhance recovery, and foster a greater sense of balance and health. Understanding how massage and mindfulness can address specific health issues helps in leveraging their benefits effectively.

Chronic Stress and Anxiety are pervasive issues that can significantly impact physical and mental health. Regular massage therapy helps to lower cortisol levels, the stress hormone, and induces a state of relaxation by stimulating the parasympathetic nervous system. This stress reduction can alleviate symptoms of anxiety, improve mood, and enhance overall emotional resilience. Complementing massage with mindfulness practices, such as meditation and deep breathing exercises, further supports stress reduction by promoting a sense of calm and enhancing emotional regulation. Mindfulness helps individuals become more aware of their stress triggers and develop healthier responses, contributing to long-term stress management.

Muscle Tension and Pain are common concerns that can arise from physical activity, poor posture, or stress. Massage therapy is particularly effective in addressing muscle tension and pain by improving circulation, relieving muscle knots, and enhancing flexibility. Techniques such as deep tissue massage and myofascial release target specific areas of tension, providing relief and promoting muscle recovery. Mindfulness practices, such as body scan meditation, can also aid in managing muscle pain by increasing body awareness and helping individuals identify and address areas of discomfort. By focusing on the present moment and tuning into physical sensations, individuals can better understand and manage their pain.

Sleep Disorders are another common health concern that can be alleviated with massage and mindfulness. Massage therapy promotes relaxation and reduces muscle tension, which can improve sleep quality and help address insomnia. By creating a calm and restful environment, massage prepares the body for sleep and supports a more restful night. Mindfulness techniques, such as guided meditation and mindful breathing, can further enhance sleep by calming the mind and reducing racing thoughts that often interfere with sleep. Establishing a pre-sleep mindfulness routine helps signal to the body that it is time to wind down, contributing to improved sleep patterns.

Digestive Issues can also benefit from the integration of massage and mindfulness. Abdominal massage techniques can improve digestive function by stimulating the abdominal organs, enhancing peristalsis, and reducing bloating. This type of massage promotes relaxation and supports the body's natural digestive processes. Complementing abdominal massage with mindfulness practices, such as mindful eating and meditation, can further support digestive health. Mindful eating encourages individuals to pay attention to their food and eating habits, which can improve digestion and reduce symptoms of gastrointestinal distress.

Chronic Fatigue and Low Energy are concerns that can be addressed through the combined effects of massage and mindfulness. Massage therapy can alleviate symptoms of chronic fatigue by improving circulation, reducing muscle tension, and promoting relaxation. This increased relaxation and improved blood flow contribute to higher energy levels and overall vitality. Mindfulness practices, such as meditation and mindful movement, help individuals manage fatigue by promoting a balanced approach to activity and rest. By becoming more aware of their energy levels and setting intentional rest periods, individuals can better manage chronic fatigue and enhance their overall sense of well-being.

In summary, addressing common health concerns with massage and mindfulness involves understanding how these practices can alleviate stress, muscle tension, sleep disorders, digestive issues, and fatigue. Massage therapy provides physical relief and enhances recovery, while mindfulness supports emotional and mental well-being, contributing to a comprehensive approach to health. By integrating these practices into daily routines, individuals can manage symptoms more effectively and foster a greater sense of balance and health.

7.1 Managing Stress, Anxiety, and Depression

Managing stress, anxiety, and depression is crucial for maintaining overall mental and emotional well-being. Integrating massage therapy and mindfulness practices offers a holistic approach to addressing these common issues, providing relief, and promoting mental health. Each practice contributes uniquely to alleviating symptoms and fostering a sense of balance and calm.

Massage therapy plays a significant role in managing stress and anxiety. Through various techniques, such as Swedish massage, deep tissue massage, and trigger point therapy, massage helps to reduce muscle tension, enhance circulation, and stimulate the release of endorphins— natural chemicals in the body that promote feelings of well-being. The physical relaxation achieved through massage therapy directly impacts the nervous system, reducing cortisol levels, which are associated with stress. This reduction in cortisol helps to alleviate anxiety, improve mood, and promote a sense of relaxation. Regular massage sessions can create a cumulative effect, leading to long-term stress relief and a more balanced emotional state.

Mindfulness practices complement the benefits of massage therapy by addressing the cognitive and emotional aspects of stress, anxiety, and depression. Mindfulness involves being fully present in the moment and observing thoughts, feelings, and sensations without judgment. This practice helps individuals become more aware of their stressors and develop healthier responses. Techniques such as mindfulness meditation and deep breathing exercises can reduce anxiety by calming the mind and promoting relaxation. Through meditation, individuals learn to observe their thoughts and feelings without becoming overwhelmed by them, which can diminish the intensity of anxiety and contribute to a more balanced emotional state.

Mindfulness-based cognitive therapy (MBCT) is a specific approach that combines mindfulness practices with cognitive therapy principles. MBCT helps individuals recognize and change negative thought patterns that contribute to anxiety and depression. By incorporating mindfulness techniques, individuals learn to interrupt cycles of rumination and self-criticism, fostering a more compassionate and balanced perspective. This approach can be particularly effective for individuals experiencing recurrent depression or chronic anxiety, providing tools to manage symptoms and improve overall mental health.

Breathing exercises are another valuable mindfulness technique for managing stress and anxiety. Deep, diaphragmatic breathing helps to activate the body's parasympathetic nervous system, which promotes relaxation and reduces the physiological effects of stress. By focusing on slow, deep breaths, individuals can calm their minds and body, reducing feelings of anxiety and tension. This practice can be easily integrated into daily routines and used as a tool for immediate relief during stressful situations.

Progressive muscle relaxation (PMR) is a technique that involves systematically tensing and then relaxing different muscle groups in the body. This practice helps individuals become more aware of physical tension and promotes relaxation. By combining PMR with mindfulness, individuals can enhance their ability to recognize and release areas of tension associated with stress and anxiety. This approach not only improves physical relaxation but also contributes to emotional well-being.

Creating a mindful routine that incorporates both massage therapy and mindfulness practices can offer long-term benefits for managing stress, anxiety, and depression. Regular massage sessions, combined with daily mindfulness practices such as meditation, deep breathing, and mindful movement, support ongoing emotional balance and resilience. By developing a consistent routine that addresses both the physical and mental aspects of stress, individuals can achieve a more comprehensive and sustainable approach to managing their well-being.

In summary, managing stress, anxiety, and depression involves integrating massage therapy and mindfulness practices to address both the physical and emotional aspects of these conditions. Massage therapy provides physical relaxation and reduces cortisol levels, while mindfulness practices promote mental clarity, emotional regulation, and stress reduction. By combining these approaches, individuals can achieve a more balanced and effective strategy for managing their mental health and enhancing overall well-being.

7.2 Relieving Chronic Pain and Muscle Tension

Chronic pain and muscle tension are prevalent issues that can significantly impact quality of life. Addressing these concerns requires a comprehensive approach that integrates both physical and mental strategies. Massage therapy and mindfulness practices offer effective methods for alleviating chronic pain and muscle tension, promoting relief, and improving overall well-being.

Massage therapy is a proven technique for relieving chronic pain and muscle tension. By applying various techniques such as deep tissue massage, myofascial release, and trigger point therapy, massage helps to target and alleviate areas of muscle tightness and discomfort. Deep tissue massage focuses on the deeper layers of muscle and connective tissue, breaking up adhesions and relieving chronic tension. Myofascial release targets the fascia, the connective tissue surrounding muscles, to release tightness and improve flexibility. Trigger point therapy addresses specific points of tension within muscles that contribute to pain and discomfort. These techniques improve circulation, reduce muscle knots, and enhance overall muscle function, leading to significant pain relief and reduced tension.

Mindfulness practices complement massage therapy by addressing the mental and emotional aspects of chronic pain and muscle tension. Mindfulness involves being present in the moment and observing physical sensations, thoughts, and emotions without judgment. This practice helps individuals develop a greater awareness of their pain and tension, allowing them to manage their responses more effectively. Techniques such as mindfulness meditation and body scan meditation can help individuals become more attuned to their body's signals, identify areas of tension, and cultivate a sense of acceptance and relaxation.

Mindfulness-based stress reduction (MBSR) is a structured program that combines mindfulness practices with techniques for managing pain and stress. MBSR teaches individuals how to use mindfulness meditation, gentle yoga, and body awareness to cope with chronic pain and muscle tension. By focusing on the present moment and developing a non-reactive awareness of pain, individuals can reduce their perception of discomfort and enhance their ability to cope with pain-related stress. This approach helps to break the cycle of pain and tension, promoting a more balanced and resilient response to chronic discomfort.

Breathing exercises are another essential component of managing chronic pain and muscle tension. Deep, diaphragmatic breathing helps to activate the body's relaxation response, reducing muscle tension and promoting a sense of calm. By focusing on slow, deep breaths, individuals can decrease the physiological effects of pain and tension, helping to alleviate symptoms. Breathing exercises can be practiced in conjunction with massage therapy to enhance relaxation and support overall pain management.

Progressive muscle relaxation (PMR) is a technique that involves systematically tensing and then relaxing different muscle groups in the body. This practice helps individuals become more aware of areas of tension and promotes overall muscle relaxation. By combining PMR with mindfulness, individuals can enhance their ability to release physical tension and manage chronic pain more effectively. This approach not only addresses muscle tension but also supports emotional well-being by reducing stress and promoting relaxation.

Creating a holistic routine that incorporates both massage therapy and mindfulness practices can provide comprehensive relief from chronic pain and muscle tension. Regular massage sessions, combined with daily mindfulness practices such as meditation, deep breathing, and progressive muscle relaxation, offer a well-rounded approach to managing symptoms and enhancing overall quality of life. By addressing both the physical and mental aspects of pain and tension, individuals can achieve more sustainable and effective relief.

In summary, relieving chronic pain and muscle tension involves a combination of massage therapy and mindfulness practices. Massage therapy provides physical relief by targeting muscle tightness and improving circulation, while mindfulness practices address the mental and emotional aspects of pain. By integrating these approaches into a comprehensive routine, individuals can achieve significant relief and improve their overall well-being.

7.3 Improving Sleep and Overall Quality of Life

Improving sleep and overall quality of life involves addressing both physical and mental aspects of well-being. Massage therapy and mindfulness practices offer effective strategies for enhancing sleep quality and fostering a more balanced and fulfilling life. By integrating these practices, individuals can experience significant improvements in their sleep patterns and overall sense of well-being.

Massage therapy is an effective approach to improving sleep quality by promoting relaxation and reducing physical discomfort. Various massage techniques, such as Swedish massage and aromatherapy massage, help to alleviate muscle tension, reduce stress, and enhance overall relaxation. By stimulating the parasympathetic nervous system, massage therapy helps to lower cortisol levels and increase the production of serotonin and melatonin—hormones that regulate sleep. Regular massage sessions can create a cumulative effect, leading to more consistent and restful sleep over time. Additionally, incorporating relaxing massage techniques into a nightly routine can help signal to the body that it is time to wind down, creating a more conducive environment for sleep.

Mindfulness practices play a complementary role in improving sleep and enhancing overall quality of life. Mindfulness meditation, which involves focusing on the present moment and observing thoughts and sensations without judgment, can be particularly beneficial for addressing sleep issues. By practicing mindfulness before bedtime, individuals can calm their minds, reduce racing thoughts, and create a sense of relaxation that supports better sleep. Guided meditation and progressive relaxation techniques can also help individuals release physical tension and prepare for restful sleep.

Mindfulness-based stress reduction (MBSR) is a structured program that combines mindfulness meditation with techniques for managing stress and improving overall well-being. MBSR helps individuals develop a more balanced stress response, which can have a positive impact on sleep quality. By fostering a greater awareness of stress triggers and promoting relaxation, MBSR can contribute to more restful and uninterrupted sleep. This approach also supports overall quality of life by enhancing emotional resilience and promoting a more positive outlook.

Breathing exercises are another valuable mindfulness technique for improving sleep and overall well-being. Deep, diaphragmatic breathing helps to activate the body's relaxation response, reducing stress and calming the nervous system. By practicing deep breathing exercises before bedtime, individuals can lower their heart rate, ease muscle tension, and create a sense of calm that supports better sleep. Incorporating breathing exercises into a nightly routine can help establish a relaxing pre-sleep ritual that promotes a more restful and restorative sleep.

Creating a mindful evening routine that incorporates both massage therapy and mindfulness practices can further enhance sleep quality and overall well-being. This routine might include activities such as a relaxing massage, mindful breathing, and meditation before bedtime. By establishing a consistent pre-sleep routine, individuals can signal to their bodies that it is time to wind down, leading to improved sleep quality and a more balanced lifestyle. Additionally, practicing mindfulness throughout the day can help manage stress, improve mood, and enhance overall quality of life by fostering a greater sense of presence and well-being.

Addressing lifestyle factors that impact sleep and overall quality of life is also important. Maintaining a healthy diet, engaging in regular physical activity, and managing stress through mindfulness and self-care practices contribute to better sleep and a more fulfilling life. By integrating these elements into a balanced routine, individuals can support their physical and mental health, leading to improved sleep and overall well-being.

In summary, improving sleep and overall quality of life involves a combination of massage therapy and mindfulness practices. Massage therapy promotes relaxation and reduces physical discomfort, while mindfulness practices support mental calm and emotional resilience. By incorporating these practices into a holistic routine and addressing lifestyle factors, individuals can achieve better sleep, enhanced well-being, and a more fulfilling life.

Chapter 8: Building a Personalized Wellness Plan

Building a personalized wellness plan is a crucial step in achieving and maintaining optimal health and well-being. A tailored wellness plan considers individual needs, preferences, and goals, integrating various practices and strategies to support overall wellness. By creating a plan that aligns with personal health objectives, individuals can enhance their quality of life and foster a balanced and sustainable approach to health.

Identifying Personal Health Goals is the first step in developing a personalized wellness plan. These goals may encompass various aspects of well-being, such as improving physical fitness, managing stress, enhancing mental clarity, or addressing specific health concerns. Reflecting on one's current health status, lifestyle, and areas for improvement helps to establish clear and achievable objectives. Setting specific, measurable, and realistic goals provides a foundation for the wellness plan, ensuring that it is tailored to individual needs and aspirations.

Assessing Current Health and Lifestyle is essential for creating a personalized wellness plan. This assessment involves evaluating existing health conditions, lifestyle habits, and areas of concern. It may include a review of dietary patterns, physical activity levels, sleep quality, and stress management techniques. Understanding these factors helps to identify areas where changes or improvements are needed. For instance, if muscle tension and chronic stress are prominent issues, incorporating massage therapy and mindfulness practices into the plan may be beneficial. Similarly, if sleep disturbances are a concern, focusing on relaxation techniques and creating a restful evening routine can support better sleep.

Incorporating Massage Therapy and Mindfulness Practices into the wellness plan can address various health goals and concerns. Massage therapy can be included as a regular practice to manage stress, alleviate muscle tension, and promote relaxation. Different types of massage, such as Swedish, deep tissue, or aromatherapy, can be selected based on individual preferences and needs. Mindfulness practices, including meditation, breathing exercises, and mindful movement, can be integrated to enhance emotional well-being, reduce stress, and improve mental clarity. Establishing a regular schedule for these practices ensures consistency and supports long-term benefits.

Creating a Balanced Routine that includes massage therapy, mindfulness, and other wellness practices is essential for achieving overall well-being. The routine should reflect individual preferences and fit into daily life. For example, incorporating a daily mindfulness meditation session, weekly massage therapy appointments, and regular physical activity can create a comprehensive approach to wellness. Balancing these practices with other lifestyle factors, such as healthy eating and adequate hydration, contributes to a holistic and sustainable wellness plan.

Monitoring Progress and Making Adjustments is an ongoing aspect of a personalized wellness plan. Regularly evaluating progress toward health goals helps to identify what is working well and what may need adjustment. Keeping a journal or using a wellness app can assist in tracking changes in physical health, mental well-being, and overall satisfaction with the plan. Based on this feedback, adjustments can be made to optimize the plan and address any emerging needs or challenges. Flexibility and adaptability are key components of a successful wellness plan, allowing individuals to make necessary changes and continue progressing toward their health goals.

Seeking Professional Guidance may also be beneficial when building a personalized wellness plan. Consulting with healthcare providers, such as a physician, nutritionist, or mental health professional, can provide valuable insights and recommendations. Professionals can offer personalized advice, help identify underlying health issues, and ensure that the wellness plan is safe and effective.

In summary, building a personalized wellness plan involves identifying health goals, assessing current lifestyle factors, and integrating practices such as massage therapy and mindfulness. Creating a balanced routine, monitoring progress, and making adjustments are crucial for achieving optimal well-being. By tailoring the wellness plan to individual needs and preferences, individuals can enhance their health, manage stress, and improve their overall quality of life.

8.1 Assessing Your Individual Needs and Goals

Assessing your individual needs and goals is a fundamental step in creating an effective and personalized wellness plan. This process involves a thorough evaluation of your current health status, lifestyle habits, and personal aspirations to develop a plan that addresses your unique requirements and supports your overall well-being.

The first step in this assessment is reflecting on your current health status. This involves taking stock of any existing health conditions, symptoms, or concerns that may influence your wellness plan. For instance, if you experience chronic pain, stress, or sleep disturbances, these issues should be identified and considered when setting goals and selecting appropriate wellness practices. Understanding your health status helps to tailor interventions and ensure that the wellness plan is aligned with your specific needs.

Evaluating your lifestyle habits is another crucial aspect of the assessment process. This includes reviewing your daily routines related to diet, physical activity, sleep, and stress management. Consider your eating patterns, level of physical exercise, sleep quality, and current methods for managing stress. Identifying areas where your habits may be lacking or contributing to health issues allows you to set realistic and targeted goals. For example, if you notice that you have poor sleep hygiene or irregular physical activity, these areas can become focal points for improvement in your wellness plan.

Identifying your personal goals is essential for creating a wellness plan that resonates with you and supports your overall aspirations. Your goals may encompass various aspects of well-being, such as improving physical fitness, reducing stress, enhancing mental clarity, or achieving better sleep. Reflect on what you hope to achieve and why these goals are important to you. Setting clear, specific, and achievable goals provides direction and motivation for your wellness plan. For instance, if reducing stress is a primary goal, incorporating mindfulness practices and regular massage therapy can be effective strategies to consider.

Considering your preferences and constraints is important for developing a plan that is both enjoyable and feasible. Think about what types of wellness practices you are interested in and how they fit into your daily routine. For example, if you enjoy relaxation techniques but have a busy schedule, you may prefer shorter, more focused mindfulness practices or self-massage techniques that can be easily integrated into your day. Additionally, take into account any constraints such as time limitations, financial considerations, or access to resources when designing your wellness plan.

Seeking feedback and support can enhance the assessment process. Consulting with healthcare professionals, such as a physician, nutritionist, or mental health counselor, can provide valuable insights and help you identify specific needs or areas for improvement. Professionals can offer personalized recommendations based on your health status and goals, ensuring that your wellness plan is safe and effective. Additionally, seeking support from friends or family can provide encouragement and accountability, helping you stay committed to your goals.

Reviewing and refining your goals periodically is an important part of the assessment process. As you progress with your wellness plan, regularly evaluating your goals and adjusting them as needed ensures that your plan remains relevant and effective. Reflect on any changes in your health, lifestyle, or personal aspirations and make adjustments to your goals and practices accordingly.

In summary, assessing your individual needs and goals involves evaluating your current health status, lifestyle habits, personal aspirations, and preferences. By reflecting on these factors and seeking professional guidance, you can develop a personalized wellness plan that addresses your unique requirements and supports your overall well-being. This thorough assessment process lays the foundation for creating a plan that is both effective and sustainable, ultimately enhancing your quality of life.

8.2 Designing a Custom Wellness Plan with Massage and Mindfulness

Designing a custom wellness plan that integrates massage and mindfulness involves creating a tailored approach to address individual health needs and goals. This personalized plan aims to enhance overall well-being by combining physical relaxation techniques with mental and emotional strategies. By thoughtfully incorporating both practices, individuals can achieve a balanced and comprehensive approach to wellness.

The first step in designing a custom wellness plan is establishing clear objectives based on personal needs and goals. This involves determining what you aim to achieve through the integration of massage and mindfulness. Objectives might include reducing stress, alleviating muscle tension, improving sleep, or enhancing emotional resilience.

Defining specific, measurable goals provides a clear direction for your wellness plan and helps in selecting appropriate practices and techniques.

Selecting appropriate massage techniques is a key component of the plan. Massage therapy offers various approaches, each with unique benefits. For example, if muscle tension and chronic pain are primary concerns, deep tissue massage or myofascial release might be suitable options. For overall relaxation and stress relief, Swedish massage or aromatherapy massage could be more appropriate. Consider your personal preferences and any specific health conditions when choosing the type of massage that best aligns with your needs. Incorporating regular massage sessions into your routine—whether weekly, bi-weekly, or as needed—ensures ongoing support for your wellness goals.

Integrating mindfulness practices into your wellness plan complements the physical benefits of massage by addressing mental and emotional well-being. Mindfulness practices such as meditation, deep breathing exercises, and body scan meditation can help manage stress, improve mental clarity, and enhance emotional resilience. Choose mindfulness techniques that resonate with you and fit into your daily routine. For example, incorporating a short daily meditation session or practicing mindful breathing during moments of stress can be effective ways to integrate mindfulness into your life.

Creating a balanced schedule for both massage and mindfulness practices is crucial for achieving optimal results. Consider how these practices can be seamlessly incorporated into your weekly routine. For instance, you might schedule a massage session once a week and dedicate a few minutes each day to mindfulness meditation or breathing exercises. Balancing these practices with other aspects of your life, such as work, exercise, and social activities, helps ensure that your wellness plan is sustainable and manageable.

Tracking progress and adjusting the plan is an ongoing aspect of your wellness journey. Regularly assess how well the massage and mindfulness practices are meeting your goals and supporting your overall well-being. Keeping a journal or using a wellness app can help you monitor changes in stress levels, muscle tension, sleep quality, and emotional resilience. Based on this feedback, make any necessary adjustments to your plan, such as altering the frequency of massage sessions or exploring new mindfulness techniques. Flexibility and adaptability are key to maintaining a wellness plan that continues to meet your evolving needs.

Incorporating lifestyle factors into your wellness plan enhances its effectiveness. Ensure that your plan includes other elements of a healthy lifestyle, such as a balanced diet, regular physical activity, and adequate hydration. These factors work synergistically with massage and mindfulness to support overall well-being. For example, combining mindful eating practices with regular exercise can complement the benefits of massage therapy and mindfulness, leading to a more holistic approach to health.

In summary, designing a custom wellness plan with massage and mindfulness involves establishing clear objectives, selecting appropriate massage techniques, integrating mindfulness practices, and creating a balanced schedule. Regularly tracking progress and incorporating lifestyle factors ensures that the plan is effective and sustainable. By tailoring your wellness plan to your individual needs and goals, you can achieve a balanced approach to health that enhances your overall well-being.

8.3 Resources and Tools for Ongoing Support and Growth

Maintaining and advancing a wellness plan requires access to resources and tools that support continuous improvement and adaptation. Whether you're integrating massage therapy and mindfulness into your routine or seeking overall health enhancement, having the right resources at your disposal can make a significant difference in achieving long-term success and growth.

Educational resources are essential for understanding and enhancing your wellness practices. Books, online articles, and reputable websites provide valuable information about massage techniques, mindfulness practices, and their benefits. Educational resources can help you stay informed about the latest developments in wellness and offer practical guidance on how to apply various techniques effectively. For example, reading books on mindfulness can deepen your understanding of meditation practices, while exploring articles on massage therapy can introduce you to new techniques and approaches.

Online courses and workshops offer structured learning opportunities to expand your knowledge and skills in massage therapy and mindfulness. Many organizations and platforms provide courses led by experts in these fields. Participating in online workshops or courses can enhance your understanding of advanced techniques, improve your practice, and provide you with new tools for managing stress and improving well-being. These educational experiences can also offer certifications or credentials that validate your commitment to wellness and help you stay motivated.

Apps and digital tools are valuable resources for integrating mindfulness and massage into your daily routine. Mindfulness apps often include guided meditations, breathing exercises, and progress tracking features that can support your practice and help you stay consistent. Massage therapy apps may provide instructional videos, self-massage techniques, and reminders for regular practice. Additionally, wellness tracking apps can help you monitor your progress, set goals, and assess the impact of your practices on your overall health.

Support networks and communities provide social support and encouragement as you work towards your wellness goals. Online forums, social media groups, and local wellness communities can connect you with like-minded individuals who share similar interests and challenges. Engaging with these networks allows you to exchange experiences, seek advice, and gain inspiration from others who are on a similar journey. Support from peers and mentors can offer valuable insights and motivation, making it easier to stay committed to your wellness plan.

Professional guidance is another crucial resource for ongoing support and growth. Regular consultations with healthcare professionals, such as massage therapists, mindfulness coaches, or mental health practitioners, can provide personalized advice and ensure that your wellness plan remains effective and safe. Professionals can help you address specific health concerns, offer tailored recommendations, and adjust your plan based on your progress and evolving needs.

Journaling and self-reflection tools are effective for tracking your progress and understanding your experiences. Keeping a wellness journal allows you to document your observations, emotions, and changes in your health over time. This practice helps you identify patterns, assess the impact of your wellness practices, and make informed adjustments to your plan. Reflecting on your experiences and setting regular check-ins with yourself can enhance your self-awareness and support your ongoing growth.

Resource libraries and toolkits provided by wellness organizations and practitioners can offer additional support. These libraries may include downloadable guides, templates, and checklists for creating and maintaining a wellness plan. Toolkits often provide practical resources that make it easier to incorporate massage and mindfulness practices into your routine.

In summary, leveraging educational resources, online courses, apps, support networks, professional guidance, and self-reflection tools is essential for ongoing support and growth in your wellness journey. By utilizing these resources effectively, you can enhance your understanding, stay motivated, and continuously improve your wellness plan, ultimately achieving lasting health and well-being.

Conclusion

As we conclude this comprehensive guide on "Massage and Mindfulness: A Comprehensive Guide to Wellness through the Body-Mind Connection and Integrating Massage and Mindfulness for Holistic Health," it is clear that the journey towards optimal well-being involves a harmonious integration of physical and mental practices. By understanding and embracing the profound connection between the body and mind, we can unlock the potential for enhanced health and a more balanced life.

Massage therapy and mindfulness, though distinct in their methodologies, converge on a shared goal: fostering holistic wellness. Massage therapy offers tangible benefits by relieving muscle tension, improving circulation, and promoting relaxation. Its various techniques, from Swedish to deep tissue, cater to different needs and preferences, providing physical relief and comfort. Through regular sessions, individuals can experience a reduction in stress and an improvement in overall quality of life.

Mindfulness, on the other hand, provides a mental framework for managing stress, enhancing emotional resilience, and fostering a deeper awareness of the present moment. By incorporating practices such as meditation, mindful breathing, and body awareness, individuals can cultivate a state of calm, improve mental clarity, and develop a more compassionate approach to themselves and their circumstances. Mindfulness practices complement massage therapy by addressing the psychological aspects of well-being, creating a comprehensive approach to health.

Integrating these two practices into a personalized wellness plan involves a thoughtful and strategic approach. Assessing your individual needs and goals is the first step in creating a plan that aligns with your specific health objectives. By selecting appropriate massage techniques and mindfulness practices, you can develop a routine that addresses both physical and mental health concerns. Establishing a balanced schedule and regularly tracking progress ensures that your plan remains effective and adaptable to your evolving needs.

The journey to wellness is not a destination but a continuous process of growth and self-discovery. Utilizing resources such as educational materials, online courses, apps, support networks, and professional guidance can provide ongoing support and enhance your ability to achieve and maintain well-being. Embracing a mindset of self-care and reflection will help you navigate challenges, celebrate successes, and continually refine your wellness plan.

As you move forward, remember that the integration of massage and mindfulness is a dynamic and evolving practice. It is not about achieving perfection but about making consistent, meaningful choices that contribute to your overall health and happiness. By nurturing both your body and mind, you create a foundation for a more fulfilling and balanced life.

In closing, this guide serves as an invitation to embark on a journey of holistic wellness, where the body-mind connection is celebrated and nurtured. By incorporating massage therapy and mindfulness into your daily life, you embrace a path of self-care that honors your unique needs and supports your journey toward a healthier, more harmonious existence.